Essential Oils
For Beginners

Use The Power Of Essential Oils & Aromatherapy For Healthy Living

Steven Ballinger

1: Introduction to Aromatherapy

2: Benefits of Aromatherapy Explained

3: Safety and Storage Guidelines

4: Aromatherapy and Weight Loss

5: How Essential Oils Can Help You Lose Weight

6: Essential Oils for Weight Loss and Metabolism

7: Suppress Your Appetite with Aromatherapy

8: Lose Weight: Change Your Mood

9: What Do Studies Say About Essential Oils?

10: How to Ensure that You Get Good Quality Essential Oils

11: Finding a Good and Qualified Aromatherapy Practitioner

12: Questions Regarding Aromatherapy and Essential Oils

13: Do-It-Yourself Essential Oil Blends

Legal Disclaimer

Introduction

As more and more Americans are becoming aware of the risks that come with being overweight, weight loss programs and diet menu plans have never been in great demand as they are today. However, there are people who can't seem to get the right formula to lose excess weight even though they've tried everything. This book is for them and for all those who simply want to lose weight.

"Ultimate Guide to Weight Loss: How to Lose Weight Using Essential Oils & Aromatherapy" will give you tips on how you can lose weight with the use of essential oils and aromatherapy. You will also learn more about aromatherapy and its benefits as well as how to make your own oil combinations.

1: Introduction to Aromatherapy

Obesity and other weight loss issues are said to be the price many Americans (as well as people in other Western cultures, for that matter) pay to enjoy a life characterized by convenience. In our desire to enjoy great-tasting meals and snacks that are prepared in less time, we often resort to processed foods lacking in—if not totally devoid of—essential nutrients.

To make matters worse, these foods are replete with all sorts of unhealthy additives, some of which are designed to make them taste better and be more filling. Couple the regular intake of such foods with a lack of exercise (Because who has the time to do that anyway?) and you have the issue of weight gain as well as the risks associated with it.

This has led to scientists, medical experts, desperate health-conscious people, and those in the health and fitness industry (who, of course, want to profit from this newfound opportunity) to come up with various practical solutions to the weight loss dilemma.

We now see drugs, medical procedures, and diet and exercise plans left and right and all promising weight loss. Many have proven to be effective, but the costs of such options and their accompanying risks have precluded their being accepted by a wider segment of the market. Still others are not convinced and instead devote their time looking for solutions elsewhere.

If you're in need of a weight loss solution and you've been hearing about—and have probably already grown tired of—the drugs, procedures, and diet and exercise plans all touted by the mainstream media as precisely what you need, here's something you probably never expected to be included in that selection: aromatherapy.

Now you may be wondering how essential oils can aid in addressing your weight loss woes. Use of essential oils is relatively simple especially when compared to the more "traditional" means of weight loss wherein certain prerequisites must be in place and specific steps have to be followed.

It has also been proven that these traditional means also work only in some cases, so what makes a much simpler option like aromatherapy effective in providing the benefits that all the other treatment options have failed to deliver? Worry not for this book will explain everything, but before all that, let's conduct a brief review of this therapeutic approach that has been in use for centuries.

Enter aromatherapy

By definition, aromatherapy is an alternative medicine which makes use of essential oils and aromatic plant compounds. The treatment's main purpose is to improve a patient's mood and overall health, primarily by inducing relaxation. Aromatherapy still has not seen widespread use, partly because some observers are skeptical about it for the simple reason that it has no scientific basis.

Remarkably, however, it continues to become more popular as more people are coming out to attest to its effectiveness in ensuring calmer bodies and minds. This is a big deal for a lot of people as many of today's commercially available drugs cannot provide the same calming effects that essential oils can. In some cases, the use of such drugs can even bring more harm than good to users.

Recent studies reveal that aromatherapy treatment does make one feel good, though there is yet to be solid scientific evidence that it can actually cure or treat any illness. Still, it must be acknowledged that such therapy is a godsend, because although aromatherapy cannot completely get rid of what ails us, it is a safe option and it can make our condition more manageable. It is possible for one to be sick without being miserable.

The principle behind aromatherapy

You may not have realized it, but different types of traditional therapies that utilize essential oils are, in effect, using aromatherapy. For instance, a massage therapist may resort to essential oils to help a client experience deep relaxation.

This alternative treatment is based on the theory that the part of the brain connected to the sense of smell is stimulated when you inhale essential oils and aromatic plant compounds. The olfactory system in the brain sends a signal to the limbic system, which is the part of the brain that controls emotions and retrieves memories. The brain releases different chemicals during the process of communication between the olfactory and the limbic systems, and this in turn helps relax and calm the patient.

Experts also say that essential oils have a direct pharmacological effect whereas proponents of aromatherapy claim that there is a synergy between the human body and aromatic oils. But scientific evidence has yet to be presented. Nevertheless, some initial clinical researches concur with this principle.

Other benefits of aromatherapy

Inhaling essential oils brings different psychological and physical effects, the first positive effect already being discussed above. On the other hand, when inhaled, the naturally occurring chemicals present in certain essential oils provide other therapeutic benefits. For instance, eucalyptus essential oil is ideal for easing nasal congestion when you have a cold. Topical application is also possible because the skin can absorb essential oils rather quickly, and thus their effects are felt much sooner. When topically applied, these oils can help in addressing beauty, hygiene, and health conditions.

Indeed, these oils derived from plant extracts have been serving various purposes since they were first discovered by ancient civilizations, and their use isn't just limited to the realm of health and beauty. This will be discussed in detail in the next chapter.

2: Benefits of Aromatherapy Explained

More and more people are favoring holistic therapy that promises to give recipients excellent benefits for the mind, body, and spirit. Fortunately for those looking for such benefits, aromatherapy promises precisely that, plus a bit more (Read: much cheaper).

Practitioners of aromatherapy affirm this holistic treatment is a combination of both creativity and technical knowledge. You need creativity to learn about the characteristics of the different essential oils and in creating new combinations. You will also need a bit of technical (scientific) knowledge to make sure that the essential oils that you use will have no adverse effects on your body.

The last thing anyone wants is therapy that is more risky than beneficial, which is one of the reasons why some people choose this and other natural treatment options over commercially available drugs and invasive surgery.

How essential oils work the mind

Essential oils came from the juice extracted from the stems, leaves, roots, or any other parts of a plant, which then undergo a distillation process. Despite being designated as "oils", there is nothing "oily" about them at all. Most essential oils are clear, but you can also find some that have a slightly yellow or amber tinge in them.

These oils are highly concentrated and have a lot of uses, but they are not to be mistaken for fragrance oils. Essential oils are derivatives of plants while fragrance oils are usually artificially made and do not have therapeutic benefits.

The aroma from essential oils stimulates the part of the brain that controls emotions. A molecule found in essential oils is like a key that will open the lock-like structures found in the olfactory nerve receptors found in your nostrils. The sensation sends messages to the limbic system in your brain. The limbic system is the central storage of your past memories, emotions, and pleasure.

Once the limbic system is stimulated, it instantly releases chemicals to the central nervous system. Some of the released chemicals, like serotonin and endorphins, eliminate anxiety and helps in reducing pain respectively. Endorphins are also responsible for an individual's response to any sexual stimulation.

Once you inhale the scent of the essential oils, you immediately enhance your whole physical and mental well-being. For instance, by placing 2 to 5 drops of chamomile essential oil on your hankie, and holding it right up your nose and then taking a deep breath, you will instantly feel relaxed.

You may also use an aromatherapy lamp, a nifty little knick knack composed of a small basin that holds a combination of water and essential oil, and a small candle (or heating element) underneath it to help diffuse the aroma of the oil throughout an entire room.

Working into the body

Besides inhalation, essential oils are also easily absorbed through the skin. The essential oils will enter the sebaceous glands and combine with the natural emollients of the skin. The chemical reaction can tone, balance, cleanse, or even deodorize the body.

Essential oils are used for their healing effects in massage therapy, body baths, foot baths, and facial steams. The essential oils are diluted with carrier vegetable oil, like sweet almond, body product, or bath water.

For instance, you can put a few drops of grapefruit oil into your warm bath and soak your body to relieve stress and muscle pain. You can also use lavender oil for cleansing and deodorizing, and it also helps revitalize dry, dull skin.

Cleanse the spirit and restore balance

Essential oils are also a staple for meditation and deep relaxation. Frankincense is not exclusively just for church services; people have actually been using it for centuries to aid in their meditation. The rich aroma of frankincense deeply penetrates the lungs, thus helping regulate your breathing so you can achieve deep relaxation and calmness when you meditate.

Essential oils have been used for many centuries because of their positive effects on the human body's overall well-being.

Essential Oils: Methods of use

These essential oils are highly concentrated compounds that need to be handled with utmost care to avoid allergic reactions. Here are some of the most common ways on how they are used:

- ***Massage***

  A therapeutic massage is one means of enjoying an aromatherapy treatment. The healing and relaxing properties of essential oils are easily absorbed when the oils are massaged into the skin. With every stroke of the therapist's hands, the body is both stimulated and relaxed at the same time, thus giving physical and emotional benefits to a recipient. A person's touch already has healing properties, and this is further enhanced with the use of essential oils.

  A massage also helps improve blood circulation and helps in cleansing out the toxins from the body, thereby improving overall well-being.

  A combination of about 3 to 5 drops essential oils and 10ml carrier oil could make good massage oil that is suitable for adults.

- ***Moisturizing Agents***

Instead of purchasing expensive skin care products, you can make your own body moisturizer and facial cream. The good thing about essential oils is they do not contain harmful chemicals and toxins that can cause allergic reactions.

The skin care products you make yourself also won't have artificial fragrances like most commercially available ones because essential oils have natural scents. They will also be free from sulphates and parabens.

Here's an example of a skin care product you can make: mix a 50g body lotion with body cream and Vitamin E cream, and just add about 20 drops of essential oil of your choice.

- ***For bathing***

  You can add about 10 drops essential to a foam base and use it as foam bath or shampoo. You can also add a few drops directly into a tub filled with warm water and soak away your fatigue, boost your energy, and uplift your mood.

- ***Perfume***

You don't need to buy expensive perfumes that have artificial colors and fragrances. You can add about 20 drops of essential oils to Jojoba oil (40ml) and you have a sweet scented perfume perfect for aromatherapy. You can also make an 80ml solution of equal parts of alcohol and rose water and add in 12 drops essential oils. Be sure to shake the bottle well and you can already use your special aromatherapy perfume.

- *Using oil burner/diffuser*

With the use of a burner or diffuser, you can fill a room with the aromatic scent of the essential oil of your choice. Add 6 drops essential oil to a candle burner/diffuser, light the candle and wait for the oil to evaporate and produce a sweet scent.

- *Fragrance spray*

Take a regular spray bottle and add cold water and 10 to 15 drops essential oil, shake well, and spray all around the room to refresh the air.

- *By inhalation*

This is the most common way of using essential oils. Take a hankie or a tissue paper, add about 1 to 2 drops of essential oils, and place it over your mouth then inhale. You can bring a small bottle of essential oil with you everywhere you go so you can de-stress yourself whenever you need to.

- *Compress*

You can also use essential oils to relieve muscle and joint pains. Just get a bowl or basin of warm or cold water and add in 4 to 5 drops essential oil. Simply soak a clean cloth and apply on the affected area.

3: Safety and Storage Guidelines

Aromatherapy is generally accepted as one the safest treatment options available. Because essential oils are derived from nature, they possess no potentially harmful synthetic additives. Still, it doesn't mean you can handle these substances any way you want.

It is imperative that you use essential oils properly to ensure your safety. They are concentrated compounds and are quite potent, which is why you need to handle them with utmost caution. For clarifying any issues and/or concerns you may have about using them or the possible effects of mishandling, you need to consult a qualified aromatherapy practitioner or a physician.

While this book was written to be a comprehensive guide for anyone just starting out with aromatherapy, it is still essential to consult with a certified professional to make sure you get the promised benefits and you guarantee your safety at the same time.

The following guidelines might be helpful:

- Essential oils must not be taken internally.

- Make sure that the oils do not come in contact with your eyes and mucus membranes. If they do, immediately wash off clean with water.

- Essential oils are not to be used by pregnant women, especially during their first trimester. It is advisable to consult your doctor first before using essential oils.

- Likewise, if you have been diagnosed with epilepsy, liver diseases, and high blood pressure, you have to consult your doctor before using essential oils. In fact, it is important that you first consult with a doctor even if you have not been previously diagnosed with any medical disorders.

- If you have allergies, make sure that you conduct the patch test first before attempting have aromatherapy treatment.

- Should you experience adverse reaction to essential oils, immediately discontinue use and seek medical attention.

- If you are using citrus oil, it is advisable that you do not expose your skin to direct sunlight.

You need to consult with your doctor if you have the following conditions but you are nonetheless set on using essential oils for aromatherapy:

- Epilepsy
- High or low blood pressure
- Diabetes
- Pregnancy
- Drinks alcohol regularly

Proper Storage

These essential oils are extracted from plants so they have a limited shelf life. Their condition will deteriorate over time and may cause allergic reactions when mishandled. To ensure that the oils' effectiveness does not deteriorate too quickly, they have to be stored in accordance with the following guidelines:

- Store your essential oils in dark glass bottles, typically amber-colored bottles.

- Keep the bottles in an upright position and at room temperature.

- Keep the bottles away from direct sunlight.

- As these oils are highly flammable, you shouldn't use them while you are near an open flame. They may also cause corrosion of plastic, rubber, and polished surfaces.

- Keep these out of reach of children and pets.

- Carrier oils also have to be handled with great care. They are also supposed to be kept away from direct sunlight and areas of your home where the temperature often fluctuates such as the kitchen and the bathroom. Their bottle caps have to be kept tightly sealed. Some practitioners recommend that the carrier oils be placed inside the refrigerator where the temperature is constantly regulated to slow down their deterioration.

Carrier Oils

The last guideline in the list provided above may have dropped a big one on you because, as a beginner, you have probably been expecting that this book would discuss only essential oils (The title may have already given you an idea.). Actually, carrier oils also fulfill a crucial role if one wishes to practice aromatherapy. Although essential oils are the key ingredient in this form of therapy as it is their potency that promotes and ensures a user's mood and well-being, many essential oils cannot be used safely unless carrier oils were used as well.

Carrier oils are so named because they "carry" essential oils and thus make it easier and safer for the latter oils to be applied to the skin. They are also known as fixed oils because they do not evaporate upon exposure to light and heat. Like essential oils, carrier oils are also extracted from natural sources such as plants, vegetables, flowers, seeds, and nuts. One factor that distinguishes them from essential oils is their very "light" smell.

Carrier oils have varying properties. They are cold-pressed, have high vitamin content, and are considered to be pure oils. They are generally used as skin conditioners. You can use them on their own or blend them with other carrier oils.

The bottom line: the majority of essential oils cannot be used safely unless these have been diluted by carrier oils first. Otherwise, you put yourself at risk of skin irritation and allergic reactions due to essential oils' strong potency.

4: Aromatherapy and Weight Loss

Over the last few years, essential oils and aromatherapy have been linked to weight loss. Studies conducted at the Niigata University School of Medicine in Japan pointed out that the body's ability to burn fat while suppressing weight gain could be activated by the scents of certain essential oils. This is especially true in the case of grapefruit and lemon essential oils, though there are other aromatic oils that can be used to aid in one's weight loss endeavors.

Before we proceed, we must first establish that essential oils are not miracle drugs that can help you lose weight instantly. If you rely mainly on them without making the necessary adjustments in your current lifestyle, especially in your eating habits and in your physical activities, then you are still doomed to fail. On the other hand, the proper use of these aromatic oils in conjunction with a proper diet and increased physical activity can be a huge help in your quest to shed those unwanted pounds.

If you want to lose weight, the first step should be determining the type of weight loss program you will undertake. It is best to consult first with a doctor to make sure that it is safe for you to do strenuous workouts or undergo dietary changes. Your doctor can also recommend a good nutritionist so you can get proper guidance on how to eat healthier.

More often than not, unhealthy eating habits and lack of physical activities cause obesity. Crash dieting is not a long-term solution to obesity. Once you have decided that you are ready to turn your life around, then you can begin considering a weight loss plan as well as the essential oils you can use in accordance with this plan.

Aromatherapy can help in your weight loss journey in many ways, such as helping curb your appetite and calming you during anxiety attack so that you don't resort to binge eating. It can even replenish your energy during workouts.

In other words, essential oils do not really ensure weight loss; rather, they *influence* it. The next chapter fully explains why.

5: How Essential Oils Can Help You Lose Weight

By now, your curiosity may be getting unbearable. Worry not, dear reader, for it is now the right time for us to discuss the specifics. This is not to say that the previous chapters are to be disregarded, though. Aromatherapy is a practice that must be done right in order for it to be both safe and effective regardless of the purpose it will serve. Hence, everything that has been discussed up to this point will serve you well as you finally go about practicing aromatherapy by yourself in the comfort of your own home.

Consultation with an expert on the matter is still important, but having the necessary knowledge can give you an advantage as you spend more time properly preparing essential oils for your weight loss needs and less time researching and asking for help just to make sure you're doing everything right.

Essential oils and weight loss

It is important to reiterate that effective and long term weight loss will not happen if you do not make changes in your eating habits and your unhealthy lifestyle. Using essential oils and aromatherapy alone will not do the trick! Safe and effective weight loss involves a multi-pronged approach using the different resources at your disposal. Relying on only one approach, like say, dieting and not resorting to exercise, won't give you the results you want within a reasonable time, if at all.

There are essential oils that can help control your appetite, make you feel confident about your own body, relieve tension and anxiety, and give you the energy boost that you need during workout sessions. As mentioned earlier, when you are actively working on a weight loss plan, you can use aromatherapy together with your diet menu plan, exercise routines, and an overall healthy lifestyle. It is important to point out that aromatherapy helps harmonize and balance your body, mind, and soul to prepare you for the weight loss process as opposed to actually causing you to shed unwanted pounds.

Essential oils can actually help shape your body with the use of the so-called multi-tiered approach:

- Essential oils from orange, grapefruit, rosemary, and cedar wood help eliminate toxins and excess fluids from your system.

- Rosemary, cardamom, and peppermint essential oils help energize your mind so that you don't skip your workout sessions.

- Essential oils like clary sage, ylang-ylang, and litsea cubeb give you positive energy and help boost your self-esteem so that you feel good about your body image. When you are recharged, there is no need for you to binge on comfort foods just to kick-start your confidence.

- Essential oils help curb your food cravings. Examples of oils that are most ideal for this purpose are fennel, spearmint, and grapefruit essential oils. They help stimulate your hypothalamus, the center of hunger in the brain, so that it neutralizes any urge to resort to comfort eating. Aromatherapy practitioners recommend that dieters carry essential oils wherever they go as such substances will come in handy at the most opportune times. For instance, should you feel the need to eat or crave something unhealthy before your next meal; you can simply open a bottle and sniff the aromatic oil contained within to suppress your cravings.

- Essential oils also help rid your body of toxins, fats, and excess fluids. Essential oils like cedar wood, orange, and rosemary have detoxifying properties that enhance the lymphatic flow to help eliminate these toxic wastes.

- Essential oils also help you change your mind so that you don't feel anxious and stressed out. Stress and anxiety often cause most people to resort to binge eating. The so-called "happy oils" include lemon and bergamot essential oils.

6: Essential Oils for Weight Loss and Metabolism

Even with a dearth of solid scientific evidence, essential oils have been confirmed by many proponents of aromatherapy as ideal for a variety of purposes associated with achieving a fitter body:

- A healthy weight loss
- Enhanced metabolism
- Increased energy
- Improved self-esteem and self-acceptance
- Elevated mood

As previously mentioned, essential oils are not your cure-all agents for resolving weight loss issues. You simply incorporate the use of essential oils so that the otherwise difficult and easy-to-abandon activities of the entire weight loss process become more doable, perhaps even more enjoyable (This will be explained in detail in Chapter 8.).

Aromatherapy is a holistic approach for ensuring that you lose weight and achieve an overall excellent health condition. Remember that weight loss involves a lot of factors: your digestive health, your lifestyle, eating habits, physical activities, diet, and stress levels. All these and the influence of your outside environment can both contribute to weight loss and weight gain.

Essential oils are often diluted with carrier oil, such as apricot kernel oil, sweet almond oil, and grapeseed oil. The resulting blended product is then applied to the skin or inhaled. They are usually available in tiny bottles. The price varies according to the country of origin of the plant source, the rarity of the plant, the quality standards of the distiller, and the amount of oil produced.

The succeeding chapters will give you detailed explanations, effective tips, and strategies on how to properly use essential oils and aromatherapy to lose weight.

7: Suppress Your Appetite with Aromatherapy

Achieving an ideal weight has always been a challenge for many people, but with plenty of tools readily available, the challenge will become less daunting. If you are among those people who have always faced that challenge, you must also keep in mind that miracle cures don't exist. Weight loss involves a sustained effort regardless of your chosen approach. Even with the aid of aromatherapy, you can't exert maximum effort only once and then expect your desired results to manifest later on.

Aromatherapy can help achieve and maintain your ideal weight

You already know that the essential oils target the special mechanisms in your brain that can help you lose weight; this is the ventro-medial nucleus of your brain's hypothalamus. It regulates your basic drives, such as your emotions and sex drive. Signals that you are already satisfied from eating are sent to the hypothalamus so that you'll stop eating. The nose is directly connected to the hypothalamus, and this is the reason why you immediately feel hunger pangs even when you merely smell food.

The essential oils that will help curb your appetite work on the same principle. When you inhale the odor molecules from the aromatic oils, they move through the mucous membrane until they reach the olfactory nerves. The olfactory nerves are receptors that take all odor molecules and intensify them so that the brain can respond accordingly.

The limbic lobe is the seat of emotions, when it activates your hypothalamus, you will feel an emotional state that triggers either a desire for food or the feeling of being full. So when you inhale the essential oils, your hypothalamus will be activated and will send signal that you are not hungry.

The hypothalamus is the seat of emotions. It alters your irrational response to food when the scent of the essential oils reaches that area of the brain. When this happens, you are basically endowed with the "power" to resist the urge to eat even if it's not yet the "right" time to eat.

Tests conducted at the Smell and Taste Treatment and Research Institute of Chicago revealed that inhalation of aromatic oil throughout the day can actually help inhibit one's food cravings. The more that people used aromatherapy to curb their appetite, the more excess weight they lost.

Aromatherapy practitioners say that the best strategy is to use different kinds of oil so that you can prevent being desensitized to the scent that will reduce the effects. With so many different essential oils that could help in weight loss, you will always have something to fall back on once you feel yourself getting used to a particular oil's scent.

What you should do

Variety in the essential oils that you use is the key to successfully control your appetite with aromatherapy. Experiment with at least three essential oils. The more you inhale those scents, the more they become effective. Be sure to change the essential oils you used the day before into a different set of three scents with each new day.

There is a special type of aromatherapy pendant used for this purpose; most of the essential oils that you can buy come with it. You just put a couple of drops onto the cotton wick of the pendant and the aroma will linger around you wherever you go. If you want a stronger scent, you can bring the aromatherapy pendant closer to your nose.

Here are some of the most recommended essential oils that can help control your food cravings:

- **Peppermint**

  Peppermint is one of the most commonly used essential oils for weight loss. It helps treat digestive problems and ease upset stomach. It is also good for weight loss. When inhaled, peppermint sends a message to the hypothalamus that you are full after every meal. This will in turn minimize your cravings so you eat less and less as the days go by. You can either inhale peppermint before eating or put a few drops in your tea or glass of water. Make sure that the peppermint you will add to your water or tea has been marked as GRAS, or generally regarded safe.

- **Grapefruit**

  Grapefruit has long been known as an effective appetite suppressant. It causes a process called lipolysis that will help dissolve excess fats in your body.

- **Bergamot**

Bergamot helps stimulate your endocrine system so that you become calm and relaxed to relieve stress and anxiety. Bergamot is known for its calming effect and it can become more potent when used together with lavender.

- *Tangerine*

Tangerine is an excellent diuretic. It can help induce calmness in your nervous system so you don't become anxious and tense, thus preventing unnecessary binge eating.

- *Orange*

Orange is also has good calming effects, and can help alleviate certain symptoms of depression.

- *Ylang-ylang*

Ylang-ylang is often used to help you clear your mind with negative thoughts. It promotes calmness and relaxation to the user.

- *Patchouli*

Patchouli is an excellent sedative. It is also used to relax tensed muscles.

Aromatherapy practitioners recommend that for your initial use; choose peppermint oil because of its unique benefits for weight loss.

Although they are more often associated with massage therapy, essential oils can actually help influence the way your body thinks about hunger and food so that you can curb your appetite. If you are unsure as to what essential oils to purchase, make sure that you consult with a qualified aromatherapy practitioner and doctor. There are oils that are not supposed to be ingested so you have to make sure that you read the labels and ask your doctor or aromatherapy practitioner for tips.

Reaching your ideal weight may not be so bad after all. With constant use, aromatherapy can help you maintain your ideal weight so that you don't get back to being obese or overweight, but that's not the only way that aromatherapy can help you get a slimmer, fitter physique. The next chapter will give you tips about how aromatherapy can change your moods in such a way that it facilitates weight loss.

8: Lose Weight by Changing Your Mood

Are you like most overweight people who eat whenever they are stressed, anxious, or bored? The danger posed by such a scenario is that an affected individual is compelled to do just about *anything* to rid himself of "that nagging feeling." Binge eating is one of the most common ways by which people try to overcome their negative moods.

It is also the least gruesome, especially when you consider the reality that some people mistakenly believe self-harm and suicide are also means of getting themselves out of the dumps. Still, obesity and being overweight are serious conditions that need to be addressed as soon as possible. Although these conditions are not really deadly by themselves, ignoring the long-term health risks associated with them could ultimately prove fatal.

It is normal to feel down at times, but luckily, there are other things that you can do to lift your spirits up besides eating, and one of them is aromatherapy. Just remember that everything actually starts in the mind; your fullness, hunger, and cravings are no exceptions. The dilemma begins in the mind. On the other hand, when you have a "healthy" mind, you begin to lose weight.

You can use aromatherapy to change your mood and relieve stress so that you don't immediately turn to food for comfort. Physically, aromatherapy can also ease pains, aches, and burns as well as help eliminate cellulite. While the results are not instantaneous, losing weight will become less difficult because you nip your hunger pangs before they become too strong to overcome.

Smell your way to a slimmer body

As discussed in an earlier chapter, recent studies have proven that there are scents that can help trigger weight loss. For instance, the mere smell of lemon and grapefruit activates your body's natural fat burning process. There is a close connection between your sense of smell and your emotions. Have you ever noticed how your mood changes when you smell something good or bad? Aromatherapy works on the same principle.

The pleasant scents from the essential oils will trigger positive reactions in your brain, and this will result in a change in your mood. When you are happy, there won't be a need for you to fill any void with food because there really isn't a void to begin with. Often, when you have nothing to do or when you're feeling down and there's no one to talk to, people resort to eating chocolates, cakes, and other sweets because these foods can trigger the production of endorphins which are the so-called "happy hormones".

There are no specific oils used for aromatherapy. It all depends on what scents will help trigger a change in your moods. One type of essential oil might work on someone you know but not on you and vice-versa. You need to experiment and try different essential oils until you arrive at the right scent. Again, consult your doctor or a licensed aromatherapy practitioner before proceeding with this approach, and remember to exercise caution when you do.

Here are some of the essential oils that can change your mood and help you lose weight:

- **To curb cravings:**

  The sweet smell of vanilla will prevent you from reaching for fattening desserts and snacks.

- **To relieve stress:**

It is best to use frankincense, jasmine, lavender, ylang-ylang, grapefruit, sandalwood, rose, benzoin, bergamot, geranium, chamomile, or vetiver. Their scents calm and relax your mind and body so you prevent feeling depressed.

- **To ease the weight of emotional baggage** that prevents you from moving forward, you can use juniper berry. Most of the time, you are being held back by the painful experiences you had in the past. When an event or a situation prevents you from enjoying your life at the present moment, you will always find something to fill that void or to at least make you forget about the past hurts, so you eat and eat. Change your frame of mind and move on, so you can begin losing weight.

- **When you need to lift your spirits up**, jasmine oil will help bring out the elusive sunshine in your life.

- **Regain confidence in yourself** by smelling essential oils made from rosemary, jasmine, orange, grapefruit, cypress, bergamot, and laurel leaves.

- *Eliminate depression* by changing your mood with these: may chang lemon, grapefruit, frankincense, clary sage, ylang-ylang, sandalwood, orange, and neroli or orange blossom. Depression is one of the main reasons why a lot of people become emotional eaters.

- *Insecurity* tends to make people withdraw socially, and when you always keep to yourself, you often see eating as a way of releasing your disappointments at your own weaknesses. Eating can make you feel good but only for a certain period only. Use these essential oils to help fight off insecurity and develop self-acceptance: jasmine, cedar wood, sand wood, bergamot, and frankincense.

- *To fight off loneliness,* try these essential oils to help ease up your negative thoughts and feelings: clary sage, rose, helichrysum, and frankincense.

- *Trigger happiness and joy* when you use orange, lemon, grapefruit, ylang-ylang, and lemon essential oils.

What You Can Do

There are different ways of using essential oils.

- **Inhale the steam**

  Inhalation is one of the most common and effective ways of using essential oils. The body's smell receptors are near the mood centers in the brain. You can add a few drops of essential oils to an oil burner or a bowl of hot water and you can inhale the aroma/steam from the oils.

- **Add to your bath**

  You can do so by combining about 6 to 10 drops of your choice of essential oil(s) and 1 tablespoon of milk into your bath. Milk will act as the carrier so that your skin won't burn as you soak your whole body onto the tub.

- **With the use of an oil burner**

  In an oil burner bowl, combine 3 to 6 drops of the essential oil of your choice with 2 tablespoon of warm water. Light the candle and wait until the pleasant aroma fills the room.

- **As massage oil**

Nothing is more relaxing and mood-changing than a soothing massage because it has both physical and emotional benefits. It is important to use carrier oil, like grape seed or almond so as not to burn your skin. Combine carrier oil (5ml) with 2 to 3 drops of essential oil.

- *A few drops on your pillow*

  You can add at least 3 drops essential oil to your pillow so you can inhale the pleasant smell as you sleep.

- *Put a few drops on your hankie*

  Your handkerchief is also a perfect tool. You can add about 3 drops of essential oil to your hankie so you can smell the scent each time you use it. It's great while you're mobile, in the office, or out grocery shopping.

Nothing should stop you from losing weight and with these practical ways of using aromatherapy and essential oils are just creative, yet simple and easy to do. Just remember that it takes proper diet and exercise, coupled with the use of aromatherapy, to lose weight and effectively maintain your ideal weight.

Additional Scents to Improve Your Overall Mood

- ### *Green apple*

  The pleasant smell of green apples can help curb your cravings. Try keeping a bottle handy so you can sniff through it when you feel like picking up a snack before your regular meals. It also changes your mood so you don't grab food when you are not feeling good.

- ### *Orange*

  The scent of orange can make you less anxious and allows you to stay calmer and think more positively. Add a few drops of orange scented essential oil to an oil diffuser to change the mood of your entire room.

- ### *Lavender*

  The scent of lavender helps fight through the pain. If you have a headache, sprinkle a few drops of lavender into your hankie and inhale the sweet scent to relieve your headache. Peppermint also has the same effect. You can try alternating lavender and peppermint to see what is more effective for you.

If you usually experience stomach cramps during your period, you can massage your abdomen with essential oils a week before you get your period. Mix in about 2 drops lavender oil, 1 drop rose oil, and 1 drop clary sage to an almond oil base.

9: What Do Studies Say About Essential Oils?

Aromatherapy is a word that you will mostly encounter among New Age or health and wellness establishments and paraphernalia. Most people would assume that aromatherapy is simply nothing but the simple use of fragrant candles or oils, with nothing more to add to their knowledge than that.

Arguably, this is partly due to "aromatherapy" being readily accessible in markets. Candles, oils, even perfume and other toiletries that have "aromatherapy" ingredients all contribute to the confusion and misconception of the practice.

In truth, aromatherapy is attributed as a form of alternative medicine used for the alleviation and treatment of various diseases and maladies that history dates to as far back as the ancient Greeks, Romans, Chinese, Egyptians, and Indians.

The fact that the practice was widely used by almost all of the great ancient civilizations could attest to its therapeutic claims. The touted essential oils made their way not only into medicinal items such as salves, creams, and poultices, but also in their perfumes and cosmetics, particularly for the

Egyptians. Cleopatra was believed to have been an avid practitioner of aromatherapy.

The skepticism involved with aromatherapy revolves around the hard scientific evidence of its many reported health benefits—or, more specifically, its lack thereof. While mention of the use of various oils, infusions, distillates, or absolutes exist in early medical journals such as in Dioscorides' *De Materia Medica* and in the works of the Persian polymath Avicenna, no modern scientific research has yet to prove of the curative powers of aromatherapy. Granted, researches show that aromatherapy can produce alleviative effects, such as promoting relaxation to the body and overall mood and clarity to the mind, though the effects are too similar to that of a perceived placebo effect to be considered as to have truly come from the inhalation of therapeutic scents and fragrances.

Advocates and practitioners the world over will attest to its efficacy, however, with some going so far as to claim that aromatherapy can have positive effects or even cure cancer. However, a lot of scientific studies are still needed in order to prove their real effect. Studies are being conducted in a global scale, currently studies are being done in Japan, India, Australia, Canada, the US, and even in Europe.

Who Does the Research?

There is a significant research agency that conducts thorough clinical studies on essential oils and their effects. Researchers belonging to the tobacco, cosmetics, food, and flavoring industries conduct regular tests and studies.

Psychologists have also tested and are still testing essential oils and their effects, particularly into how the essential oils are able to change the mood and emotions of an individual that can influence or override one's basic instincts and drives.

They are also interested in seeking further studies about the possible toxicity levels of these essential oils. The safety of the consumers is the foremost goal of these studies.

Most researches are not available to consumers as they are mostly proprietary. However several studies have been published in medical journals for public viewing. A few of which include studies about the effects of aromatherapy and essential oils to patients who are suffering from dementia.

Another of which is a study concerning the therapeutic use of lavender oil to treat and control anxiety. In fact, lavender oil, of which aromatherapy advocates and practitioners will claim that the mild flowery scent has a calming effect and therefore is widely used for relaxation and as an alternative solution to sleeping disorders, is an additive to an approved anxiolytic oral drug that exists and is still currently being used in Germany.

Studies have shown that lavender oil contains high amounts of linalyl acetate and linalool, which both contain anxiolytic or anti-anxiety properties.

What are the Issues or Concerns about the Studies?

Some essential oils used in aromatherapy have been researched and studied to support their medicinal use; others have not. This is particularly true to essential oils with claimed effects that are bordering on the deeper functions of the brain, such as emotion, cognition, and memory. A few studies have yielded positive results, though scientists believe that the results could be attributed more to a placebo effect rather than to the claimed therapeutic effect of the essential oils.

Scientists have some unique issues in the study of essential oils. They are as follows:

- *They are not standardized*

The chemistry of most essential oils is dependent on its location and weather conditions in the area. The time of day when the plant sources were harvested is also another factor in determining its chemical composition, so is the season during harvest time. The way they are processed, packed, and stored also has a huge influence on their chemistry.

Each plant has its own unique chemistry; hence, there are no essential oils that are exactly the same. There is a big difference between essential oils that were obtained from natural organic sources and from cultivated sources used primarily for pharmaceutical drugs.

Moreover, the essential oils themselves pose a great risk of discrepancy, as there are several parts of the plant that could be used to derive the oils, as well as the fact that there could be several types of plants within the same family.

For example, a bottle of essential lavender oil could come from one or a mixture of sources;

oils could have been derived from seeds, leaves, or flowers. Additionally, oils could be derived from different types of lavender plants, which could produce different therapeutic effects.

As there is no clear-cut standardization of how and where essential oils should be obtained, manufacturers are free to use and possibly adulterate their essential oils and still market it is "100% pure". After all, the leaves, seeds, flowers, and stalks of the lavender plant are still parts of the lavender plant, so theoretically speaking, it is still justifiable to say that the bottle of essential oil is "100% pure", even though only a fraction of which was derived from the therapeutic part.

However, they can be altered in order to achieve standardization. The problem though is that when essential oils undergo standardization process, they lose their naturally-occurring properties, which effectively cancels out the claim.

The differences in place, time, and conditions of the harvested plant pose a huge challenge to scientists conducting the studies. At present, the International Standards Organization has a set of standards that manufacturers have to follow to ensure that acceptable concentrations are produced that are safe for use of the end-users.

- ***Scientists are finding it hard to effectively conduct "blinded" studies of the aromatic substances***

A typical study involves two groups to be tested: one to get an experimental substance, while the other will get a placebo substance or substance coming from the "control" group. When it comes to aromatic substances, scientists have difficulty conducting a blinded study. Some scientists make use of masks in order to "blind" the participants during the testing.

There are still some who try using alternate scents that are known to have an absence of therapeutic properties as controls, such as ground coffee beans or coffee bean oil, which is used by perfumers and chefs to cleanse the sense of smell and rid themselves of aromatic intoxication. These strategies are difficult because people usually associate scents with past experiences, thus, it is quite difficult to clearly establish how essential oils actually affect every individual.

- ***Researchers are finding it hard to get funding and approval for their clinical studies***

Essential oils have been in existence for thousands of years and they have been used by humans since ancient times. Because of this, they don't really fit into the conventional clinical science type of testing in the laboratory, on both animals and finally in humans. Most groups have the tendency to fund those that follow the more scientific approach of researches.

Most studies done conventionally are commissioned or funded by the pharmaceutical industries themselves. However, only few companies invest in these researches because of the limited potential to profit, mainly due to the fact that these products come from natural sources and are hard to be patented.

- ***Researchers find it hard to tell the exact reason for the result***

With conventional researches, establishing the exact causes of the outcome is necessary. However, when essential oils are tested, they are often used as adjutants to other therapeutic methods, such as in the case of massage therapy, making it difficult to pinpoint which caused the positive outcome, whether from the use of essential oil or the massage itself. It is also important to point out that essential oils have hundreds of chemical constitutions, making it difficult to determine which particular constituents caused the desired effect.

What do the end results say?

Recent researches show many positive effects to a substantial amount of health issues, including chronic pain, common infections, depression, anxiety, premenstrual syndrome, vomiting, nausea, tumors, and a lot more, though extensive and conclusive clinical testing to produce hard evidence is still lacking. Be that as it may, however, aromatherapy has survived some thousands of years, and whether its efficacy is attributed to its inherent properties or to a perceived placebo effect, the fact remains that aromatherapy *does* work, to a certain degree.

10: How to Ensure that You Get Good Quality Essential Oils

The quality of the end product will only be as good as the quality of the ingredients. As a consumer (or an aromatherapy practitioner), you obviously want to get excellent quality products to obtain positive and effective results. However, because there are so many different kinds of essential oils, it is hard to assess their quality. Essential oils can come from anywhere around the world. Most retailers and suppliers get their stocks directly from farmers or wholesalers. The end users do not actually have any knowledge about the practices and the relationship between the suppliers and the farmers or wholesalers, not to mention the handling and bottling procedures by the companies. Most consumers are more concerned in the treatment of their medical issues.

If you are one of those consumers who want to know how you can ensure that you are getting excellent quality products, you will learn a lot from this chapter.

How essential oils are regulated

The FDA or Food and Drug Administration is the agency responsible in regulating foods, additives, drugs, dietary supplements, and cosmetics in America. Other countries will have similar agencies, though the scope and set of standards might differ from those of the FDA of America.

Legal classification is based on how the products are supposed to be used. The FDA classifies essential oils as drugs or cosmetics, depending on their use, preparation, and application. The agency makes classification on a case-to-case basis. For instance, if a manufacturer claims that the aromatic scent of their product (essential oil) promotes beauty, the FDA will most likely categorize their product as a cosmetic. On the other hand, if the manufacturer says that their essential oil can effectively help treat or prevent a specific medical condition, the product will be categorized as a drug. As such, different categories will warrant different regulations, so a bottle of FDA-approved cosmetic lavender oil versus a bottle of FDA-approved medicinal lavender oil might be different or not.

Drugs or Cosmetics – Is there any difference?

Drugs and cosmetics are regulated differently. While essential oils are used for therapeutic purposes (or drugs); most oils are not considered by the FDA and other agencies as drugs. Hence, they can be purchased without getting a prescription from a medical doctor. In addition, as drugs are assumed to be taken directly to the body, such as orally or topically, a stricter set of rules and standards must be met before a product receives the FDA approval.

However, cosmetics are assumed to be applied superficially, and away from sensitive areas such as the mucus membranes, therefore allowing a more flexible set of standards. Other companies might opt to pass off their essential oils as beauty products instead of medicinal supplements because of this loophole.

How is Ad Claims Regulated?

Most manufacturers make claims via their ads, but will not necessarily indicate so on their labeling. For example, a manufacturer of lemon oil might advertise their product as a possible way to reinforce or support weight loss, but will not print the same claims on the lemon oil bottle's label itself. This is most often the case in alternative medicine or supplements, which also gains attention due to the rapid exchange of information through mass media especially the Internet.

Medicinal or therapeutic claims can be posted online, with bottles or preparations of the said medicinal item claiming that there are "no approved therapeutic claims" with the usage of the said product. These claims are oftentimes used to bypass the security and testing of various food and drug administrations of different countries. If they print on their label that their product is not actually proven to produce medicinal or therapeutic effects, the possible positive or negative effects will fall entirely upon the consumer's own discretion.

In the US, the agency responsible in monitoring this aspect is the Federal Trade Commission. On the other hand, room fragrance systems, like odor control and deodorizers, are regulated by the Consumer Product Safety Commission.

There is an agency assigned in promoting the development of standardization of products on a global level. This agency is the International Organization for Standardization or ISO. The ISO provided guidelines for essential oils to cover packaging, storage, labeling, testing, sampling, and conditioning, among others.

What can Influence the Quality of Essential Oils?

There are several factors that can influence the quality of essential oils:

- **_Plants_**

  The quality of the end product will be greatly affected if the plant sources are treated with chemicals, such as pesticides. The quality is soil's variability and its conditions, such as the amount of rainfall, and the classification in terms of species and varieties, can also affect the obtained oils.

- **_Processing_**

  The use of essential oils have become popular over the years and because of that some products that are available in the market today might have little to no medicinal or therapeutic value or use due to adulteration. You can now purchase them everywhere, in retail stores, online shops, discount stores, and health food stores all over the world. Some products might be pure while others might have been diluted or have undergone unnecessary processing that compromise its quality and effectiveness. As a general rule, 100% pure, natural and organic, cold-pressed essential and carrier oils are preferred and are generally considered to be the highest grade.

- ***Handling and packaging***

  Handling, packaging, and storage are other factors that can impact the quality of essential oils. There is a possibility of chemical degradation occurring when the oils are exposed to light, heat, and oxygen. For instance, citrus-based essential oils are prone to oxidation that can possibly alter the end product's chemical composition. This is why essential oils should be contained in air-tight tinted bottles. Also, oils lose their potency over time. Bottles with a manufacture date of over two years will be less potent than freshly-bottled oils.

- ***Storage***

  Essential oils cannot be stored in typical containers. They have to be stored in dark, glass containers that are tightly closed. They have to be stored in a cool, dry place to ensure that it maintains its high quality. Manufacturers recommend writing the date on the bottle when it was opened so that monitoring it is easier. Oxidation varies for different essential oils, but most can be used for about 1 to 2 years after the bottle is opened.

Regardless of where you obtain your oils, you have to make sure that you are getting them from reputable sources to ensure that you are buying excellent quality products. The problem is that an agency that solely controls and monitors the quality of essential oils manufactured and sold to consumers is non-existent in the US. However, you can make use of the following questions to gather information about the products you are considering of purchasing, especially when buying from an online store:

- Is the Latin name of the plant source indicated? This ensures that the essential oil is obtained from the specie tested to have beneficial effects. For instance, lavender alone has several known species, while only a handful have been tested and proven effective.

- Is the country of origin of the plant source indicated in the label? While an ordinary end user (such as a consumer) would not be able to know the difference, but an experienced aromatherapy practitioner does. These practitioners are aware that the quality of the plant sources would vary by country. Oils derived from the countries home to the plants are better than in countries who only cultivated the plants.

- Is there an indication of purity? It has to be indicated whether it is 100% natural essential oil or it is a mixture of several essential oils, or if there were alterations in the chemical composition. For instance, essential oil is different from fragrance oil, as the latter is a combination of essential oils and chemical fragrances.

- Can you compare the cost with the other brands carrying the same essential oils? Most of the time, if a particular product is cheaper than similar ones, it might not be genuine or authentic. This is because some manufacturers might entice consumers with a cheaper product but at the cost of diluting the essential oils with alcohol or carrier oil.

- Does the label indicate any information about the plant source being organic or not? It is important to take note that most essentials oils that are being sold in the United States are not certified organic, however, there are

European-manufactured essential oils that are definitely organic.

You will be using these essential oils on your body so you have to ensure that you are purchasing excellent quality products. If you are unsure about what to buy, you can ask a practitioner of aromatherapy to help you with your choices.

11: Finding a Good and Qualified Aromatherapy Practitioner

You may opt to find an aromatherapy practitioner to perform the preferred treatment for you. The best way of finding a good practitioner is to ask friends and family for referrals. Some alternative clinics will have listings of qualified aromatherapy practitioners. You may also ask your healthcare provider to suggest a few names.

Aromatherapy is evident in many different traditional alternative practices, so a qualified practitioner might not be labeled as such. Practitioners and advocates of Ayurveda medicine are also knowledgeable in aromatics and essential oils, as these are also used in many aspects of traditional Indian cultures.

The same can be said of acupressure practitioners and acupuncturists, as scents are also used in meditation and in the regulation of *chi* or body energy, which is a staple principle in most Eastern alternative practices.

When you are choosing an aromatherapy practitioner, there are several factors to consider, like one's education, training, experience, and their philosophy of providing care. This might be difficult in other countries, as not all have fully embraced alternative forms of medicine as scientific practices, so practitioners and experts more or less will only cite years of experience to their claim.

However, countries like the UK and Australia have dedicated schools for the study and practice of alternative medicine, so it is still possible to find practitioners who have studied the alternative form. Ayurveda medical practitioners could hail directly from India. Subsequently, acupuncturists and acupressure practitioners could have studied from China, Singapore, and Hong Kong. It is advisable to get a short list of names to choose from. You have to choose one that you feel is suitable for you and for your specific needs.

What to expect when you go to an aroma therapist

When you work with an aromatherapy practitioner, it is like working with your doctor or any health care provider. You have to make sure that you give the practitioner all the details and information that he or she needs regarding your health.

Having all the needed information ensures that the practitioner can treat your specific needs. It is therefore important that you give the therapist the detailed information about your allergies, illnesses, chronic health conditions, and other important environmental factors. Histories of mental illness such as depression or seizures are also essential.

The practitioner should also be able to tell you of your rights and responsibilities as a client, as mandated by law. There are states that have specific statutes that are aligned with their policies and regulations, so you have to be knowledgeable of those particulars.

The actual procedure depends on the condition that you want to be treated and your response to the treatment itself. It is imperative that you pay attention to how your body is responding to the treatment because you might need to undergo follow-up sessions as the treatment continues.

If you feel like you might be experiencing negative effects, and you are just doing the treatment on your own, you have to immediately stop from using the essential oils and consult an aromatherapy practitioner. For serious medical conditions being treated with the use of aromatherapy, you have to make sure that there are other health care providers involved in the treatment. They can give you

therapies and treatments that can complement
aromatherapy.

12: Questions Regarding Aromatherapy and Essential Oils

Q: *Are essential oils safe?*

A: This is one of the most common questions people have about essential oils. Most of them are generally safe and do not have adverse side effects if they are used according to instructions. Factors to consider the essential oils' safety include:

- *Dosage*

   It is necessary that you use the right dosage to ensure your safety. Some people use too much of the potent oils. It should be stressed that essential oils should not be used directly when administering topically and should always be diluted by a carrier or base oil. A high dosage and/or concentration might cause burning of the skin or other irritations, such as in the case of tea tree oil, which is often added in facial beauty products for its astringent properties.

- *Purity*

Some manufacturers alter the composition of essential oils and add synthetic chemicals, diluting the oils with the use of vegetable oil. Always look at the labels. It is not bad if a bottle has 20% essential oil and 80% vegetable oil, especially for essential oils that are really expensive, like rose and neroli, in order to make them affordable, but try to find essential oils that are diluted in high-quality carrier oils, such as extra virgin olive oil, virgin coconut oil, jojoba oil, and other such oils. If you using high concentrated pure essential oils, you will have to dilute them for safety purposes.

- *Method of application*

There are essential oils that are best inhaled, while some are meant to be used topically as they can irritate the air passage. Never take essential oils orally. If you are unsure, you have to consult a practitioner to get tips on the proper usage.

- *Possible reactions with medications*

There might be possible reactions between some essential oils and pharmaceutical drugs. You will need to let your healthcare provider assess your condition, including your medications if you are considering getting aromatherapy treatment. For instance, oil of Wintergreen contains high amounts of methyl salicylate, which can have potentially dangerous effects to people taking anticoagulants like Warfarin, aspirin, or garlic capsules.

Q: *Is there a possibility for essential oils to be toxic?*

A: With the right amount of dosage and administration, there is a slim chance of toxicity occurring with the use of essential oils. It is important to reiterate that essential oils are not to be ingested.

Dilution is an important step when preparing the use of essential oils. As a general rule, a lower dosage should be used in children. However, there are some essential oils that are not suitable for children, like peppermint. Caution should also be exercised when using essential oils in pets.

The topic of restrictions has been discussed in earlier chapters.

No matter how essential oils are considered as safe to use, it is important that safety measures are in place. Improper use and handling can often result in unpleasant results. When in doubt, do not hesitate to consult a professional.

Q: *Do I need to go to an aroma therapist to receive optimum treatment?*

A: While it is actually your own personal preference if you want an aroma therapist to treat you, the information that you are getting from this book should be able to help you with your decision. Even if you are doing the treatment yourself, it will do you good if you will at least consult with a professional aromatherapy practitioner, just to get specific and important information such as the right dosage, proper application methods, purity, and possible interactions of the essential oils if ever you are taking medications.

The rule of the thumb is if you are in doubt, consult an experienced aromatherapy practitioner or ask assistance from a professional healthcare provider to help you.

Q: *Do aromatherapy practitioners have licenses?*

A: There is no licensure exam in the United States for the practice of aromatherapy. It is possible, though, that the aromatherapy practitioner is a licensed healthcare provider, like a nurse or physical therapist. The general practice codes for aromatherapy are: they have to demonstrate a level of training and competence, including the skills to do aromatherapy treatment. Additionally, aromatherapy might be a class or subject tackled in associated with a more complex form of alternative medicine, so an alternative medical practitioner or doctor might be knowledgeable of aromatherapy as well.

An ordinary person practicing aromatherapy doesn't have a license in the US, but these people can have more experience and training in the use of aromatherapy and essential oils than any healthcare provider. It is thus, imperative that you ask a potential practitioner of his skills, trainings, and experience.

Q: *Is there at least a certification process for aromatherapy practitioners?*

A: The US does not have a certification process or requirement for the practice of aromatherapy, but there are groups that have set their implementation programs. For instance, the National Association for Holistic Aromatherapy or NAHA is a nonprofit educational organization that has their own education guidelines for their aromatherapy training programs.

The Aromatherapy Registration Council or ARC has a registration process being offered to practitioners who exhibit core competence and knowledge about aromatherapy and essential oils if they pass the national examination. This registration serves as self-regulation for people who practice aromatherapy, though they are not required or mandated by law to file for registration. However, for a practitioner who is looking at getting more clients, an RATM or Registered Aroma therapist title after their names would be a boost to their credentials.

Q: *Is aromatherapy an expensive treatment?*

A: There is no standard cost for the treatment; it is for the practitioner or the therapeutic clinic to determine the cost of treatment. Arguably, treatments are less expensive than most conventional treatments, and different aromatherapy clinics will most likely price treatments within the same range. Included in determining the costing is the type of oil used, whether it is single or blended with other oils, the length or duration of the treatment, and if there are other requirements needed or asked for, such as massages or meditative exercises.

If you are considering of purchasing essential oils for your personal use, prices can range from under $10 for a small 10ml bottle to up to a hundred dollars for the exotic or premium-grade oils. Lavender, eucalyptus, peppermint, and tea tree oils are generally inexpensive, while pure rose oil is hard to find and is considerably more expensive.

13: Do-It-Yourself Essential Oil Blends

This last chapter will give you practical applications and easy do-it-yourself mixes of essential oils that can help you lose weight. Researches continue to further prove their effectiveness in the weight loss process. You have been given a list of essential oils that you can use to help you lose weight; here you will learn what can effectively be mixed with what to increase their potency.

Effective weight loss inhaler

This comes in handy especially when you are out or have to go to the office. Carrying a small bottle or infused potpourri packet it in your bag allows you to inhale the aromatic scent anytime you feel sugar cravings.

In small dark glass bottle or PET plastic bottle, put 1 teaspoon coarse sea salt and add any of the following essential oil blends:

Citrus Blend Aromatherapy

30 drops of grapefruit oil

4 drops of lemon oil
1 drop of ylang-ylang oil

Mint Blend Aromatherapy

20 drops of peppermint oil
10 drops of bergamot oil
4 drops of spearmint oil
1 drop of ylang-ylang oil

Herbal Blend Aromatherapy

15 drops of basil oil
15 drops of marjoram oil
1 drop of oregano oil
1 drop of thyme oil

How to use the aromatherapy inhaler

The weight loss inhaler is easy to use: simply take 3 long, low, deep breaths of the aromatic scent. Take a short break, and then take 3 more deep breaths. Do this cycle at least thrice. The best way to do it is to inhale slowly while counting to five seconds through each of your nostril. Remember, more is better, so do not hesitate to inhale as deep as you can.

You can do this 5-15 minutes before every meal or whenever you feel that you are craving for sweets or salty food in between your regular meal time. There are studies showing that it is more effective if you inhale the aroma at regular intervals throughout the day.

An ever better strategy is to change scents daily so your system does not get used to it and develop familiarity, which can cause you to plateau and render the essential oil inefficient. You have three blends here and you can prepare three bottles and alternate them each day.

Another problem that could arise from this is aromatic intoxication. This happens when the nose gets subjected to too many scents within a short period, which can result to a temporary numbing or dulled sense of smell. This problem most often occurs in people whose jobs require them to smell several product samples, such as perfumers or fragrance consultants for bath and body products.

Chefs and other food-industry workers are also at risk for aromatic intoxication, which could prove to be mildly disastrous when they taste their food. Taste is highly dependent on smell, so having a dulled olfaction will also dull the sense of gustation. They address this issue by carrying packets of ground coffee beans, or carrying a small bottle of coffee bean oil to smell in between samplings. The aroma of coffee beans cleanses the olfactory senses, countering the effects of aromatic intoxication. You could also use this trick to help your olfaction keen for essential oils.

Bonus Tips: *Aromatherapy during workouts*

When you are trying to lose weight, it is essential that you adapt healthier lifestyle and eating habits. Here are helpful tips that you can use when you are working out:

Preparing for a Workout

- Add a few drops of grapeseed essential oil to your lotion or to plain water, rosewater, or aloe vera gel. You are not supposed to topically apply undiluted essential oils directly to your skin because they are highly concentrated and might cause allergic reaction.

- Another option is to get a 4-ounce spray bottle and fill with water, and then add 7 drops each of geranium, rosemary, eucalyptus, peppermint, and palma rosa essential oils. Mix well and spritz on every exposed area of your body. Allow to dry on the skin while you drink water and doing some stretching routines as you prepare for a workout session. The listed essential oils are known for their energizing properties.

- You can still work out even if you have asthma, although a consult with a physician is still recommended. You will need concentrated massage oil composed of 10 to 30 drops eucalyptus essential oil and 1 oz of grapeseed oil. Eucalyptus oil helps dilate the air passageways and improves circulation. You can topically apply the massage oil to your throat, neck, chest, upper back, and temples.

- You can also combine 3 drops each of orange, geranium, rosemary, lavender, black pepper, and peppermint essential oils with 2 oz grapeseed oil. You can gently rub the mix onto the muscles that are likely to get sore after your workout. These oils are known to relieve muscle tension and pain.

During Workout

- You still need to stay energized when you are working out. In a spray bottle, put 3 oz water and 1 oz witch hazel oil and mix well. You may also add in 5 drops sage, 12 drops bergamot, and 7 drops of cypress essential oils. Spray on your skin as you are sweating. Spray on areas that prone to breakouts but make sure that you protect your eyes.

- You can reapply the essential oil blend you made above to soothe sore muscles. This helps in the circulation while you do stretching exercises.

Post Workout

- Topically apply diluted tea tree oil to your feet immediately after you shower. Tea tree oil has anti-microbial properties. You can dilute tea tree oil with extra virgin olive oil, virgin coconut oil, avocado oil, or jojoba oil. These oils are all moisturizing oils that will help soothe dry and cracked skin. As an added benefit, virgin coconut oil has an antifungal effect.

- Use this to massage on your sore muscles: 2 oz grapeseed oil/lotion, 20 drops clove oil, 10 drops thyme, and 20 drops eucalyptus oil.

- Have an aromatherapy diffuser at home to relieve stress and induce relaxation. Recommended scents are lavender, thyme, tea tree, and eucalyptus.

- You can also apply a blend of 10% jojoba oil and 90% *Helichrysum italicum* (everlasting oil) to strains and bruises from working. This mixture enhances circulation and speeds up the healing process.

Losing weight requires determination and dedication, and the slow process of seeing the results might dishearten most people from continuing with their regimen. A successful weight loss program needs to consider the whole body's wellness, meaning that the emotional and psychological aspects of the person should be reinforced as well.

Aromatherapy and essential oils alone will not result to weight loss, but the benefits of this ancient practice will help reinforce one's will and determination to continue. It should be noted that if the only issue is mind over matter, then reinforcing the mind will surely yield more favorable results.

Conclusion

This book has given you all the information that you need to effectively lose weight while incorporating aromatherapy and essential oils into your routine.

With the help of this book, you will discover that essential oils and aromatherapy have a lot of other uses aside from the relaxing effect you can get from spas and massage salons.

Please do not forget to share your learning with family and friends, so they too, can live a fuller and healthier life!

Thank you for downloading this book and good luck!

www.ingramcontent.com/pod-product-compliance
Lightning Source LLC
Chambersburg PA
CBHW070602290526
45790CB00002B/749